Quality Sleep and Relaxation

Quality Sleep and Relaxation:

A Comprehensive Guide for Better Sleep, Relaxation, and Happiness.

Anna P. Coburn

Dedication

To my mindful loved ones, who have everlastingly been my inspiration and my sincerely strong organization. Much obliged to you for engaging me to seek after my dreams and for ceaselessly staying nearby, during the most inconvenient times. This book is committed to you, with all my fondness and appreciation.

Chapter 1

Introduction - Explanation of the importance of good sleep and relaxation

Do you struggle with getting a good night's sleep? Do you find it hard to unwind and relax after a long day? If so, you're not alone. In today's fast-paced world, it's easy to become overwhelmed and stressed, which can take a toll on our ability to rest and rejuvenate. That's why I'm excited to share with you my new eBook, "Quality Sleep and Relaxation."

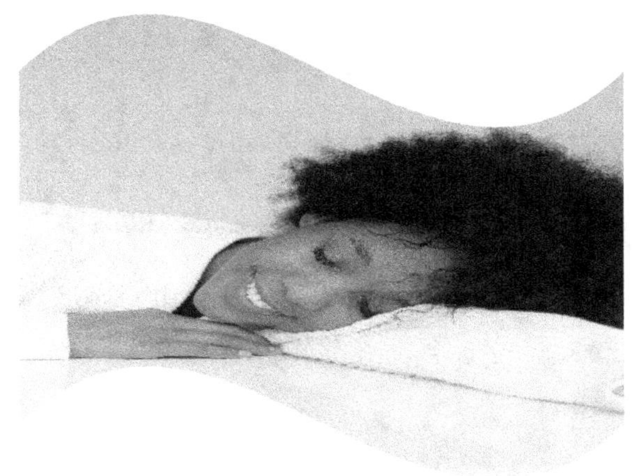

Sleep and relaxation are essential for our physical and mental health. They allow our bodies and minds to recharge and rejuvenate, preparing us for the challenges and opportunities of each new day. Unfortunately, in today's fast-paced world, it can be challenging to get the rest we need.

Lack of sleep and relaxation can lead to a range of health problems, including obesity, diabetes, cardiovascular disease, and depression. It can also impair our cognitive functioning, affecting our memory, attention, and decision-making abilities. In short, not getting enough sleep and relaxation can have serious consequences for our overall well-being.

On the other hand, getting enough quality sleep and relaxation can have a range of benefits, including improving our mood, increasing our productivity, and reducing our risk of chronic health problems. So, it's clear that making sleep and relaxation a priority in our lives is essential for maintaining our physical and mental health and achieving our goals.

Overview of meditation and mindfulness practices as tools to improve sleep and relaxation

In this eBook, you'll learn about the importance of good sleep and relaxation and how they contribute to our overall well-being. You'll also discover the power of meditation and mindfulness practices as tools to improve your sleep and relaxation. From body scan meditation to yoga, this eBook offers a range of techniques to help you relax, unwind, and get a better night's sleep.

Each chapter is designed to provide you with a comprehensive understanding of the technique, step-by-step instructions for practicing, and the benefits it offers for sleep and relaxation. Whether you're a beginner or an experienced meditator, there's something for everyone in this eBook.

So, if you're ready to take control of your sleep and relaxation and start feeling more rested and rejuvenated, I invite you to dive into

"Meditation and Mindfulness Practices for Better Sleep and Relaxation." With the right tools and techniques, you can transform your sleep and relaxation habits and improve your overall quality of life.

Chapter 2

Body Scan Meditation - Relax Your Body and Mind

Do you ever feel like you can't turn your mind off, even when you're trying to relax or sleep? Body scan meditation can help. This technique involves systematically bringing your attention to each part of your body, noticing sensations and releasing any tension or discomfort. By doing so, you can learn to relax both your body and mind.

Body scan meditation can be done lying down or sitting up, whichever is most comfortable for you. To get started, find a quiet and comfortable place where you won't be disturbed. Wear comfortable clothes and remove any distractions such as your phone or computer.

1. *Explanation of the technique*

To begin, close your eyes and take a few deep breaths. Then, bring your attention to the top of your head and notice any sensations in this area. Move slowly down your body, one body part at a time, noticing any sensations and releasing any tension or discomfort.

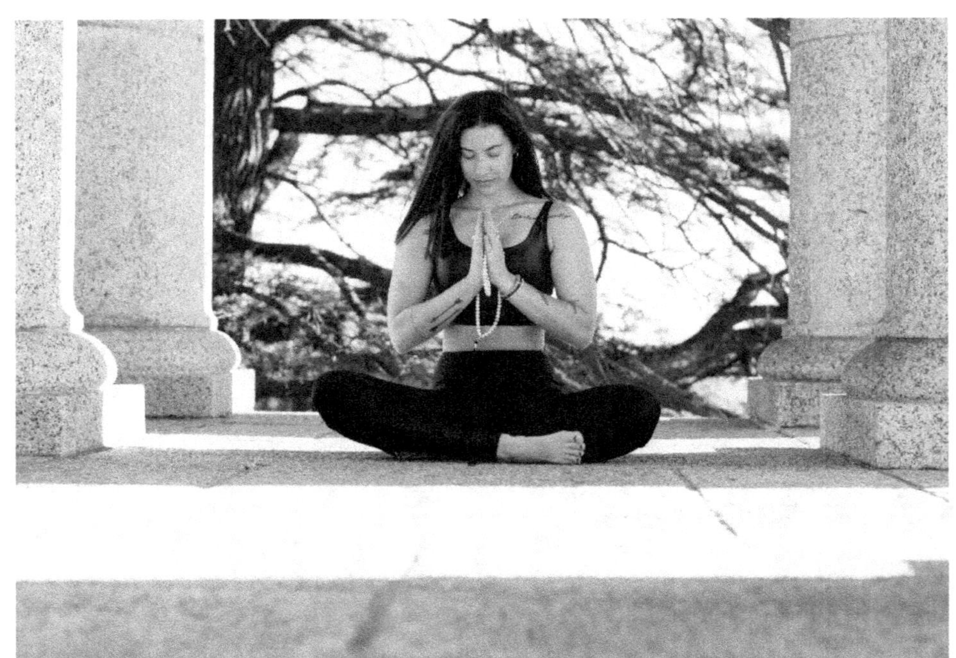

As you do this, try to focus solely on each body part, avoiding any distractions or thoughts.

2. Step-by-step instructions for practicing body scan meditation

- Start by lying down or sitting in a comfortable position.

- Take a few deep breaths and allow yourself to relax.

- Begin at the top of your head and bring your attention to this area. Notice any sensations such as tingling, warmth, or pressure. If you notice any tension or discomfort, consciously release it as you exhale.

- Move down to your forehead and notice any sensations here. Again, release any tension or discomfort as you exhale.

- Continue moving down your body, focusing on each body part one at a time. Pay attention to your eyes, cheeks, jaw, neck, shoulders, arms, hands, chest, stomach, back, hips, legs, and feet.

- As you scan each body part, notice any sensations, and release any tension or discomfort. Try to stay focused on each body part and avoid any distractions or thoughts.

- Once you have completed the body scan, take a few deep breaths and allow yourself to relax.

3. Benefits of body scan meditation for sleep and relaxation

Body scan meditation can be a powerful tool for improving sleep and relaxation. By systematically releasing tension and discomfort from each body part, you can learn to relax both your body and mind. This can help to reduce stress, anxiety, and racing thoughts that can keep you awake at night. Additionally, body scan meditation can help to improve body awareness and reduce chronic pain or discomfort. With regular practice, you may notice improvements in your sleep quality, overall relaxation, and sense of well-being.

Incorporating body scan meditation into your daily routine can help you to develop a deeper connection with your body and improve your ability to relax and sleep. Give it a try and see the benefits for yourself.

Chapter 3

Mindful Breathing - Calm Your Mind and Body with Your Breath

Have you ever found yourself feeling overwhelmed or stressed and wished you could just take a deep breath and relax? Mindful breathing is a powerful technique that can help you do just that. By focusing on your breath and observing it without judgment, you can calm your mind and reduce stress and anxiety.

Mindful breathing can be done anywhere, anytime, and in any position. To get started, find a quiet place where you won't be disturbed. Wear comfortable clothing and remove any distractions such as your phone or computer.

1. Explanation of the technique

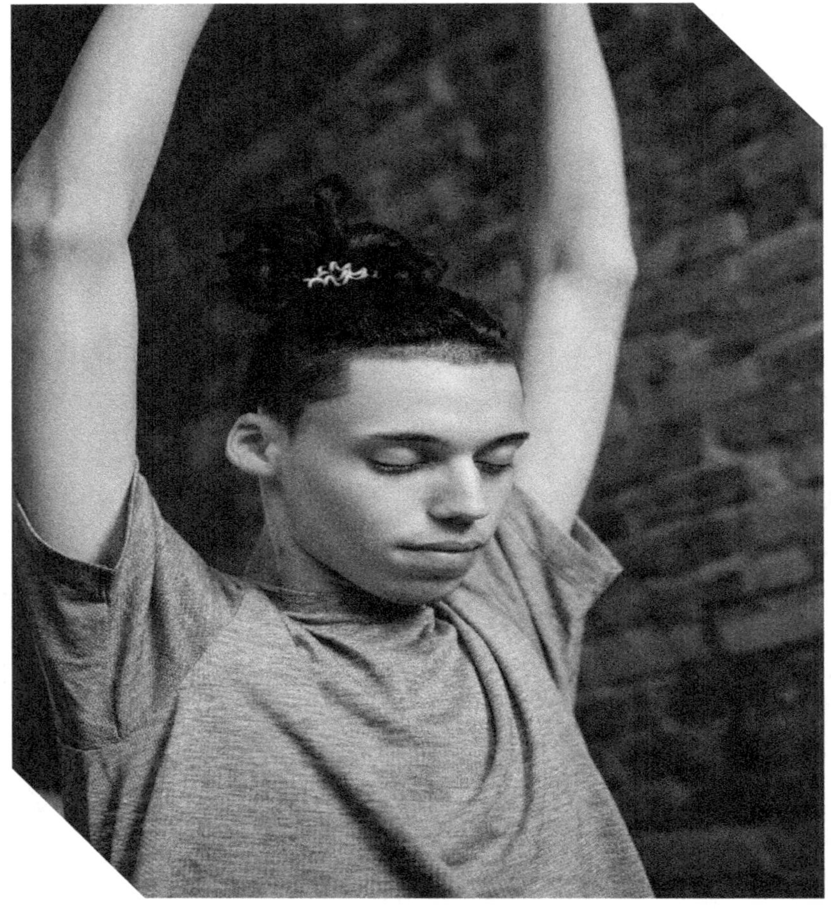

Mindful breathing involves bringing your full attention to your breath and observing it without judgment. It's a way to anchor your mind in the present moment and become more aware of your thoughts, feelings, and sensations.

2. Step-by-step instructions for practicing mindful breathing:

- Find a comfortable position, either sitting or lying down, and close your eyes.

- Take a few deep breaths and allow your body to relax.

- Bring your attention to your breath. Notice the sensation of the air moving in and out of your body.

- Observe your breath without trying to change it. Notice if it's deep or shallow, fast or slow, smooth or uneven.

- If your mind wanders, gently bring it back to your breath. Try not to judge your thoughts or become attached to them.

- Continue observing your breath for a few minutes, or as long as you like.

- When you're ready to end your practice, take a few deep breaths and bring your awareness back to your surroundings.

3. Benefits of mindful breathing for sleep and relaxation:

Mindful breathing is a simple yet powerful technique that can have numerous benefits for sleep and relaxation. By focusing on your breath and observing it without judgment, you can calm your mind and reduce stress and anxiety. This can help to lower your heart rate and blood pressure, which can lead to better sleep quality. Additionally, mindful breathing can improve your ability to concentrate and focus, which can also improve your sleep quality. With regular practice, you may notice improvements in your overall sense of well-being and your ability to relax and sleep.

Incorporating mindful breathing into your daily routine can help you to develop a deeper connection with your breath and improve your ability to relax and sleep. Give it a try and see the benefits for yourself.

Chapter 4

Guided Imagery - Relax Your Mind with Visualization

Have you ever found yourself lost in a daydream, imagining a peaceful scene or a relaxing environment? Guided imagery is a technique that can help you intentionally and systematically use your imagination to create a calming and soothing experience for your mind and body. It can be a powerful tool for improving sleep and relaxation.

Guided imagery involves creating a mental picture of a peaceful or calming environment, using all of your senses to fully immerse yourself in the experience. You can do this on your own or with the help of a recorded guided imagery session. Here's how to get started:

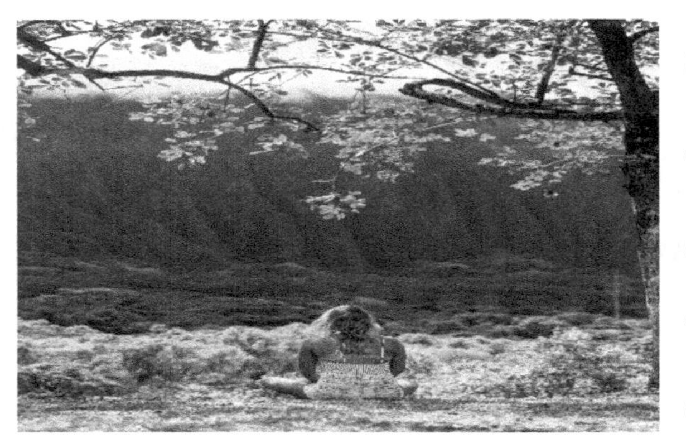

To begin, find a quiet and comfortable place where you won't be disturbed. Sit or lie down and take a few deep breaths to relax your body and mind. Then, imagine a peaceful or calming environment, such as a beach, forest, or mountainside.

Use all of your senses to fully immerse yourself in this experience. Imagine the sights, sounds, smells, textures, and tastes of this environment.

2. Step-by-step instructions for practicing guided imagery

- Find a quiet and comfortable place where you won't be disturbed.

- Sit or lie down and take a few deep breaths to relax your body and mind.

- Choose a peaceful or calming environment to imagine, such as a beach, forest, or mountainside.

- Close your eyes and use all of your senses to fully immerse yourself in this experience. Imagine the sights, sounds, smells, textures, and tastes of this environment.

- As you imagine this environment, notice any tension or discomfort in your body and consciously release it as you exhale.

- Continue to focus on this peaceful environment, allowing yourself to fully relax and let go of any stress or worries.

3. Benefits of guided imagery for sleep and relaxation

Guided imagery can be a powerful tool for improving sleep and relaxation. By creating a mental picture of a peaceful environment, you can give your mind a break from the stress and distractions of everyday life. This can help to reduce anxiety, racing thoughts, and other sleep disruptors. Additionally, guided imagery can improve mood and reduce symptoms of depression. With regular practice, you may notice improvements in your ability to relax, fall asleep, and stay asleep.

Incorporating guided imagery into your daily routine can be an effective way to reduce stress and improve your ability to relax and sleep. Whether you use a recorded session or create your own mental picture, allow yourself to fully immerse in the experience and enjoy the benefits of a calmer and more peaceful mind.

Chapter 5

The Power of Progressive Muscle Relaxation

Have you ever felt like your muscles are so tense that you can't seem to relax no matter how much you try? Progressive muscle relaxation (PMR) is a simple but effective technique that can help you release tension and achieve deep relaxation. In this chapter, we will explore what PMR is, how to practice it, and the amazing benefits it can have on your sleep and relaxation.

Explanation of the Technique

PMR is a relaxation technique that involves tensing and releasing different muscle groups in your body. By contracting and releasing each muscle group, you can become more aware of the sensations in your body and gradually release any tension you are holding. This technique was first developed by Dr. Edmund Jacobson in the early 1920s and has since been used as a stress-reducing tool in various contexts.

Step-by-Step Instructions for Practicing Guided Imagery

Here's how you can practice PMR:

1. Find a quiet and comfortable place to sit or lie down.

2. Take a few deep breaths and close your eyes.

3. Focus your attention on one muscle group at a time, starting with your toes.

4. Tense the muscle group by squeezing it as hard as you can for a few seconds.

5. Release the tension suddenly and notice the feeling of relaxation spreading through your body.

6. Move on to the next muscle group, working your way up from your feet to your head.

7. Take deep breaths throughout the exercise and focus on the sensation of relaxation in your body.

Benefits of Guided Imagery for Sleep and Relaxation

The benefits of PMR are numerous, and it has been found to be particularly effective for improving sleep and reducing anxiety. By releasing tension in your muscles, you can reduce physical discomfort and promote relaxation. PMR has also been shown to decrease symptoms of insomnia, lower blood pressure, and improve overall mood.

Incorporating PMR into your daily routine can have a profound impact on your physical and mental well-being. Whether you practice it before bed or during the day to reduce stress, PMR is a powerful tool for achieving deep relaxation and better sleep.

In conclusion, progressive muscle relaxation is a simple but effective technique that can help you release tension and achieve deep relaxation. By following the step-by-step instructions outlined in this chapter, you can begin to reap the benefits of this powerful technique and improve your sleep and relaxation.

Chapter 6

Progressive Muscle Relaxation - Ease Your Tension and Sleep Better

Do you find it difficult to relax and unwind after a stressful day? Progressive muscle relaxation may be the solution you need. This technique involves tensing and then relaxing each muscle group in your body, helping you to release physical tension and achieve a deep sense of relaxation. By doing so, you can improve your sleep quality and overall well-being.

Progressive muscle relaxation can be done in any comfortable position, such as lying down or sitting up. To get started, find a quiet and comfortable place where you won't be disturbed. Wear comfortable clothes and remove any distractions such as your phone or computer.

1. *Explanation of the technique:*

Progressive muscle relaxation is a technique that involves tensing and then relaxing each muscle group in your body.

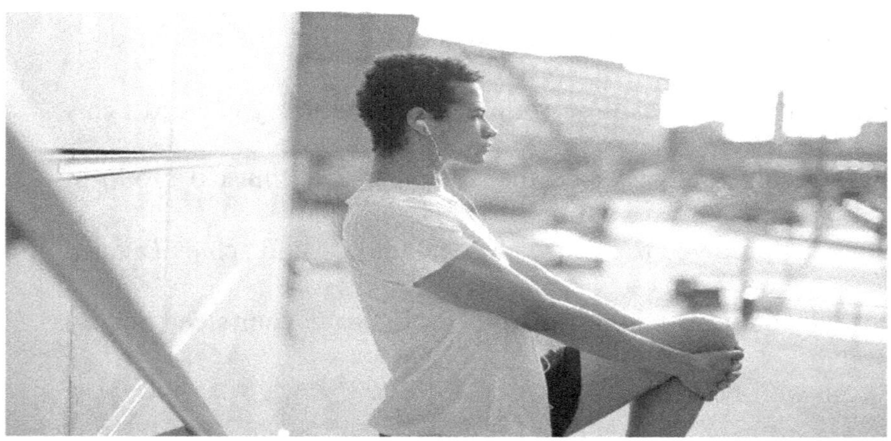

By doing so, you can release physical tension and achieve a deep sense of relaxation. This technique can help you to become more aware of your body and how it feels, and it can also help to reduce stress and anxiety.

2. Step-by-step instructions for practicing progressive muscle relaxation:

- Start by finding a comfortable position, either sitting or lying down.

- Take a few deep breaths and allow yourself to relax.

- Begin by tensing the muscles in your feet. Hold this tension for a few seconds, then release as you exhale.

- Move up to your calf muscles and repeat the process of tensing and releasing.

- Continue up your body, tensing and then releasing each muscle group in turn. Move to your thighs, hips, stomach, chest, back, arms, hands, neck, and finally your face.

- As you tense each muscle group, try to hold the tension for a few seconds, then release as you exhale. Try to focus solely on the physical sensations in each muscle group and avoid any distractions or thoughts.

- Once you have gone through each muscle group, take a few deep breaths and allow yourself to fully relax.

3. Benefits of progressive muscle relaxation for sleep and relaxation

Progressive muscle relaxation is a powerful tool for reducing physical tension and achieving deep relaxation. This technique can help to improve sleep quality, reduce stress and anxiety, and promote overall well-being. By becoming more aware of your body and how it feels, you can also learn to release tension more easily and achieve a greater sense of calmness. With regular practice, you may notice improvements in your sleep quality, overall relaxation, and sense of well-being.

Incorporating progressive muscle relaxation into your daily routine can help you to release physical tension and achieve deep relaxation, allowing you to improve your sleep quality and reduce stress and anxiety. Give it a try and see the benefits for yourself.

Chapter 7

The Power of Yoga for Sleep and Relaxation

Yoga has been used for centuries as a tool to promote relaxation and restful sleep. It combines physical movement, deep breathing, and mindfulness to calm the mind and relax the body. In this chapter, we will explore how yoga can help you achieve better sleep and relaxation, introduce you to basic yoga poses, and highlight the many benefits of incorporating yoga into your mindfulness and meditation practice.

Combining Movement, Breath, and Mindfulness

The practice of yoga is unique in that it combines physical movement, deep breathing, and mindfulness. The physical movements help to release tension in the body, increase flexibility, and improve circulation, while the deep breathing helps to calm the mind and promote relaxation. With the addition of mindfulness, the practice of yoga becomes a powerful tool for reducing stress and promoting restful sleep.

Introduction to Basic Yoga Poses for Sleep and Relaxation

Some basic yoga poses that can help promote relaxation and better sleep include:

1. Child's Pose: This gentle pose is a great way to stretch the hips, thighs, and ankles while also 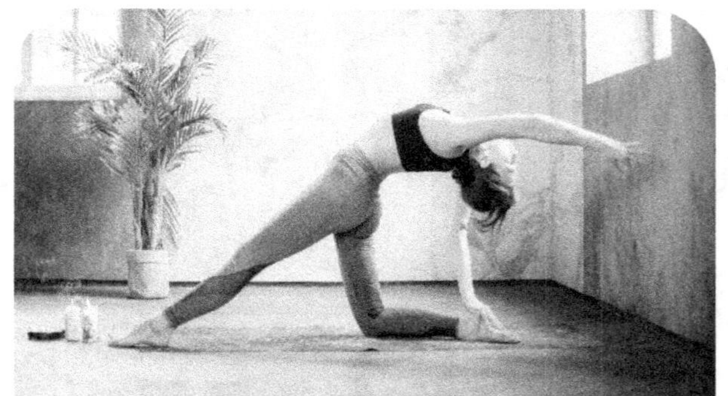

promoting relaxation and stress relief.

2. Cat/Cow Pose: This pose involves gently arching and rounding the spine while also syncing the movement with the breath. It can help to relieve tension in the back and neck while also calming the mind.

3. Forward Fold: This pose involves bending forward at the hips and letting the head and arms hang down towards the ground. It can help to release tension in the back, neck, and shoulders while also calming the mind.

Benefits of Yoga for Sleep and Relaxation

The benefits of yoga for sleep and relaxation are numerous. Regular practice can help to:

1. Reduce stress and anxiety

2. Improve sleep quality and duration

3. Increase flexibility and mobility

4. Promote overall relaxation and well-being

Incorporating yoga into your mindfulness and meditation practice can be a powerful way to promote better sleep and relaxation. By combining physical movement, deep breathing, and mindfulness, yoga can help to release tension in the body and calm the mind, creating the perfect conditions for restful sleep and relaxation.

Chapter 8

Conclusion - A Better Night's Sleep Starts with Meditation and Mindfulness

In today's fast-paced world, it's no wonder that so many people struggle with sleep and relaxation. But the good news is that you don't have to rely on medication or other interventions to get a good night's rest. By incorporating meditation and mindfulness practices into your daily routine, you can learn to relax your body and mind and get the sleep you deserve.

Throughout this eBook, we've explored various techniques, including body scan meditation, mindful breathing, guided imagery, progressive muscle relaxation, and yoga. Each of these practices has unique benefits for sleep and relaxation, and you may find that one or more of them works best for you.

Some of the benefits of meditation and mindfulness practices for sleep and relaxation include reducing stress and anxiety, improving body awareness, reducing chronic pain or discomfort, and promoting a sense of well-being. These practices can also help you to develop a deeper connection with your body and mind and improve your overall quality of life.

But the key to success with meditation and mindfulness is to find what works best for you. You may need to experiment with different techniques and approaches before you find the one that resonates with you. Remember, meditation and mindfulness are not one-size-fits-all, and what works for one person may not work for another.

So, if you're struggling with sleep or relaxation, take the time to explore the techniques outlined in this eBook. Experiment, practice regularly, and most importantly, be patient with yourself. With time and dedication, you can learn to relax your body and mind and get the restful sleep you deserve.

Congratulations! You have now learned about a variety of meditation and mindfulness practices that can help you achieve better sleep and relaxation. By practicing these techniques, you can reap a multitude of benefits, including reduced stress, increased self-awareness, and improved overall well-being.

Remember, everyone is different, and what works for one person may not work for another. That's why it's important to try out different techniques and find what works best for you. Whether it's body scan meditation, mindful breathing, guided imagery, progressive muscle relaxation, or yoga, there's a technique out there that can help you achieve better sleep and relaxation.

So, don't be afraid to experiment and try new things. With practice and patience, you can learn to incorporate these practices into your daily routine and experience the many benefits they have to offer. Sweet dreams!

Acknowledgement

I might want to offer my gratitude to my friends and family for their assistance through the imaginative cycle. Extraordinary thanks to the experts in consideration, care, and rest for their significant encounters. I in like manner thank my editor and disseminating bunch for their constant exertion. Eventually, I'm appreciative to the perusers who will benefit from this book.

www.ingramcontent.com/pod-product-compliance
Lightning Source LLC
Chambersburg PA
CBHW061532250726
48657CB00005B/2194